Home Workout:

Become Slim And Muscular in 30 Minutes a Day With 15 Best Proven Workouts

The information herein is offered for informational purposes solely, and is universal as so. The presentation of the information is without contract or any type of guarantee assurance.

The trademarks that are used are without any consent, and the publication of the trademark is without permission or backing by the trademark owner. All trademarks and brands within this book are for clarifying purposes only and are the owned by the owners themselves, not affiliated with this document.

Table of content

Introduction

Many people assume that in order to get slimmer they need to start on an extreme diet. This is something that often seems to be encouraged and endorsed by celebrities through the huge array of fad diets which appear regularly. The fact that these celebrities are generally slim seems to enforce the authenticity of the diet. However, whilst it is important to consider what you eat, undertaking an extreme diet whilst starting an exercise plan can be damaging to your health.

The biggest change you can make to your body to encourage weight loss and build your muscles is to look at the calories you consume. Reducing them to below the level of the number you consume in a day will result in weight loss. However, this weight loss can often be from water and even your muscles! This is due to the fact that, if the body does not know when it will next get food, it switches to survival mode. This means it stores fat, removes excess water and burns energy from your muscles. This is not what you are trying to achieve!

Instead you should be looking at consuming either the recommended daily amount of 2,500 calories for men and 2,200 for women or just a little more. What matters most about your diet is the balance. Protein is an important nutrient which will help to build your muscles and help them to recover after a workout. Carbohydrates are necessary but in moderation; these are the normal fuel for the body and burn slowly to provide energy for long periods of time. Sugar is one of the substances you should do your best to avoid; although even this in moderation is of benefit.

Once you have established a diet which will support your exercise regime you can focus on completing the thirty minute workouts listed in this book. They are separated into section; five workouts for beginners who are new to working out, five for the intermediate level and five for those of you who are already well on the way to improved muscles and fitness levels. You can upgrade any exercise when it suits you by simply upping the number of reps, increased the resistance or moving up a level. There is no wrong or right pace; merely the one that works best for your body and your goal.

It is also important to note that the more you use your muscles the more calories you will burn. Muscle mass has been shown to burn more calories than fat and encourages blood flow around the body; helping you to stay healthy and making you less likely to contract an array of diseases such as coronary heart disease, diabetes or even some types of cancer.

You may also be surprised at how good you feel after completing an exercise routine. Exercise releases endorphins into the blood stream; these make you feel good and give you a sense of accomplishment; this is why so many athletes appear to be addicted to exercise!

Chapter 1 – 5 Workouts for Beginners

One of the most difficult parts of exercising is motivating yourself to start and actually completing your desired amount of exercise per day. One of the best ways to approach this issue is to select a time when you will exercise; this can be first thing in the morning or last thing at night. What matters is that you set a routine and you stick to it. Once you have established a schedule you will need will power to stick to it. Many people find that keeping a picture of what you would like your body to look like can help to motivate you. It will not take long before you start to see some results and this will drive you to do more; as already mentioned it can become extremely addictive. The great thing about the following workouts is that you do not need any special equipment; they can be completed anywhere.

It is important to remember that, before any exercise, you must warm up properly. A warm up means slowly building the use of your muscles so that they warm gradually; this reduces the chance of injury and improves the results of your workout.

1. *The Body Weight Circuit*

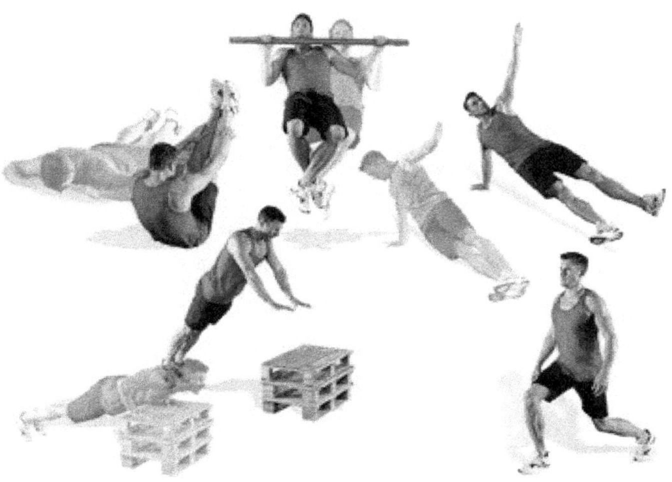

http://assets.menshealth.co.uk/main/thumbs/32319/nobell.jpg

The idea behind this routine is to complete each exercise and move straight onto the next without a break. By doing this you will improve your strength, stamina and effectively complete a cardio workout as well. The ultimate aim is to complete the following circuit three times. However, especially when you first start you are likely to get tired often. If you are too tired to complete the next exercise then stop, catch your breath and start again. It is much better to complete an exercise properly than to attempt it and injury yourself.

The first step is to do twenty body weight squats; these involve bending your legs to ninety degrees and angling your back forward at forty five degrees. You can support yourself if needed whilst building your muscles. It is similar to sitting down; without the support.

Next, you can follow this with ten push-ups and then twenty lunges.

Once these are complete you should attempt ten dumbbell rows; this means placing your right knees on a bench and bending forwards. Your chest should become parallel to the floor. You can then grip a weight on the floor with your palm facing towards you and pick the weight up; bending your arm ninety degrees before, lowering it back down after a count of five. The weight should lift above the line of the bench. After you have done ten on one side you will need to do ten on the other.

Finally you can finish with a fifteen second plank and thirty jumping jacks.

2. *Upper Body Routine*

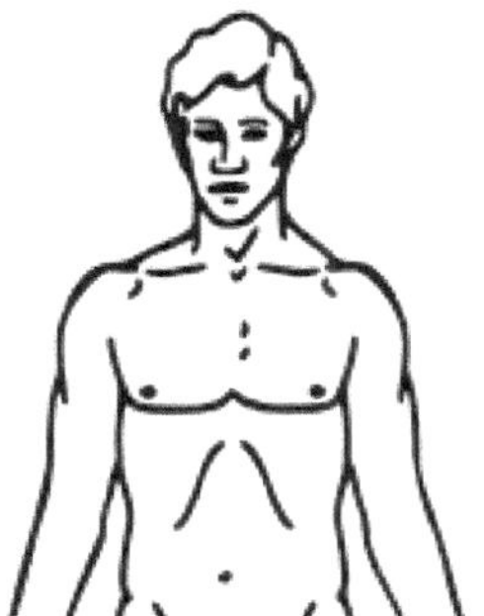

https://upload.wikimedia.org/wikipedia/commons/thumb/a/af/Pioneer_plaque_man_upper_body_as_diagram_template.svg/2000px-Pioneer_plaque_man_upper_body_as_diagram_template.svg.png

This routine, as its name suggests involves focusing on your upper board. The idea behind this is focus is to do this routine several times a week and mix other routines in. Variance has been shown to help build muscles and help to keep you motivated:

The first step is to complete between eight and twelve resistance band chest presses. This simply involves purchasing a relatively cheap resistance band and wrapping it around a solid object; roughly in line with the middle of your back. You can then grasp each end of the resistance band with your arms bent and tucked in next to you. Simply stretch them forward and then slowly back. Once you have completed your reps you can rest for one minute before doing the same again. Complete this cycle three times.

You will then need to do as many pushups as possible within twenty seconds. After a ten second rest you should repeat the push-ups until you have done this eight times.

The third step involves the military press; a weight will be required for this exercise and it literally requires it to be lifted straight up from the floor to above your shoulders. You will need to start with a comfortable weight size and move up as you build muscles. You should do as many as you can in forty seconds, pause for fifteen and repeat another two times.

Next the front and side raise involves using your weight in one hand and lifting it away from your body whilst keeping your arm straight. This should be repeated ten times with a sixty second rest before you do it twice more.

Finally, add a plank for thirty seconds, with a rest of thirty seconds before repeating the plank.

3. Legs

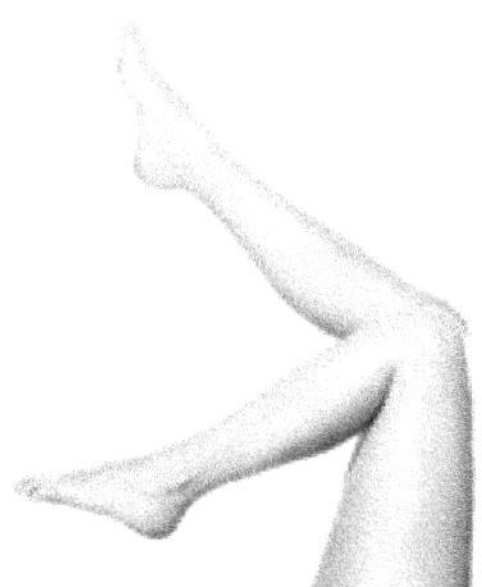

http://pngimg.com/upload/leg_PNG4792.png

It is essential to complete a balanced workout to ensure your muscles build across your body. There are too many examples of men with massive shoulders and tiny legs!

Start by completing a hip thruster; this is an excellent exercise for sculpting your buttocks and thighs. Simply lie on your back and thrust your hips into the air; hold them there for two seconds before lowering and repeating fifteen times. You can then rest for fifteen seconds before repeating the reps twice more.

The next step for your legs is to complete some step ups; these can be on a stair, bench or even a specific machine. You should do twelve reps, followed by a nine-ty second break and then another two sets of twelve.

Finally, the tuck jump can be performed five times with a rest of sixty seconds before another five and then one more set of five! Simply jump, tucking your knees into your chest and then land squarely back on your feet.

4. *The Barrel Chest*

This is to improve the muscle definition of your chest, your general strength, core and stamina. To start- with you will need a pull-up bar or a sturdy door frame that you can get a good grip on. You should place your hands on the frame and then pull yourself up until your chin is above the frame or bar, (where your hands are). The aim is to do as many of these as possible in sixty seconds. You can then complete fifteen push-ups before doing a plank for sixty seconds.

Finally, you will need to do what is known as the renegade row. This involves using two weights. Place both on the floor and ensure you have a good grip on them. Start by lifting on hand and brining the weight up to your waist; you arm should bend with your elbow behind you. Next you can lower this arm back down and repeat with the other arm; repeat this ten times.

Once you have completed the whole set, you can rest for two minutes before repeating them all. As your muscle strength grows you will be able to repeat this five times.

5. The Whole Body

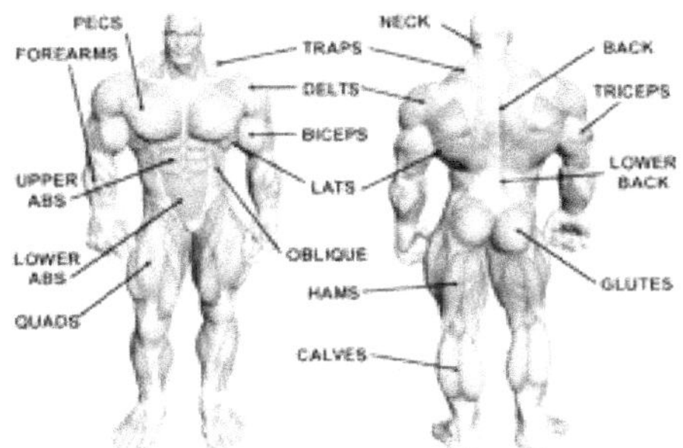

COMMON NAMES FOR MAJOR MUSCLE GROUPS

https://upload.wikimedia.org/wikipedia/commons/9/99/Body_muscles.jpg

Start by completing ten dumbbell lunges. This involves standing up straight with a dumbbell in each hand. Simply step forward and bend your front leg to ninety degrees. The back leg should do the same and be just above the ground.

Next you can do a dumbbell dead lift; simply place the dumbbells on the floor in front of you. Bend at the knees and with a straight, angled back to pick the weights up and bring them to waist height. Repeat this eight times.

You can then hold a dumbbell in your hand with your arm by your side. Bring the dumbbell up slowly to touch your shoulder; repeat ten times for each arm.

This is followed by planking for sixty seconds and then ten push-ups. The last parts of the routine involve using an AB wheel or a can of beans! Simply knee down and push the wheel or can out as far as you can in front of you. You must not let your body touch the ground before you roll back to the starting position. Repeat this exercise eight times before finishing with the dip. This involves supporting yourself on both sides; possible with sturdy chairs and lifting yourself up, with knees bent. You waist should be at the line of the bars with your arms straight. You then lower yourself down until the bars are in line with your chest. Hold for three seconds and return to the starting position. This should be repeated eight times. You can then rest for two minutes before re-doing the whole routine; ideally twice.

Chapter 2 – Five Intermediate level workouts

Once you have mastered the beginner levels you will want to move onto something more difficult. The following workouts are more challenging and will continue to build your muscles. It is possible to mix these with the beginner level workouts or even to do all of them. The important thing is to do what is most comfortable for you. Every workout should push your limits without risking injury; you will notice that your limits gradually change as your muscles improve.

1. *The No Equipment Option*

Simply follow these steps to feel the burn, improve your muscles and your cardio. Ideally this can be used to help slim and tone your existing muscles; this makes it the perfect accompaniment to a muscle routine:

Jumping jacks for two minutes should be followed by twenty side lunges. These involve doing a lunge as described earlier but to the side of your body and stretching your hands down to your foot. After you have done one side you should do the other.

Next you will need to do twenty squats; you should hold a weight in each hand and gradually increase the heaviness of this weight as your squats improve. This can be followed by skipping for two minutes; preferably with a rope.

The next step involves lying on the floor and lifting your hips into the air. As an advancement from the beginner stage you can add weights to your legs or waist using a weight belt.

It will then be time to complete some arm circles. Simply hold your arms out straight on each side with a weight in each hand. Your palms should be facing upwards. Bring each arm in to your should at the same time as squatting. This can be followed by simply holding the weights straight out at arm's length to each side for thirty seconds.

Next you will need to lie down again. Keep your knees bent and hold your weight in one hand with it resting on your shoulder; slowly lower the weight past your shoulder and onto the floor. You can then bend your legs to one side and slowly straighten your arm whilst lifting your head and shoulders off the floor. This should be repeated ten times for each side of your body.

Finally finish with ten push-ups, ten sit ups and a cross crawl; this involves raising your right knee and holding your arms in the air. Slowly lower your left elbow to your raised right knee and then repeat with the right elbow and left knee. Do this as fast as possible for two minutes.

The routine should take thirty minutes although it is likely to take longer on your first few attempts.

2. Upper Body

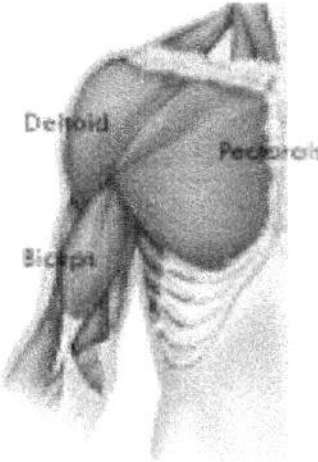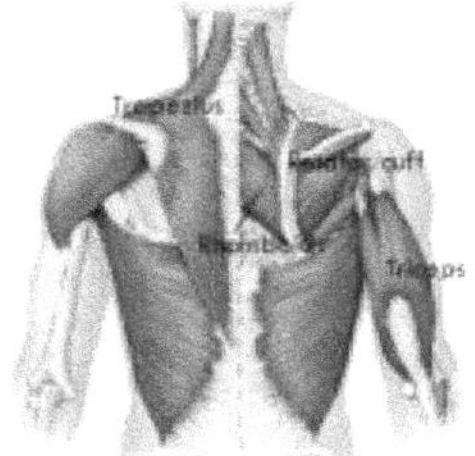

http://www.rivertea.com/blog/wp-content/uploads/2014/01/upper-body-muscles.jpg

This routine should be carried out at least three times a week alongside some of the other workouts listed in this section. Te key to becoming more muscular is to focus on every muscle group, in your body at different times. This will ensure your body develops evenly. It can also be an excellent way to provoke muscle growth as it is different to the normal routine you have been following:

You will need to do ten dumbbell bench presses, followed by ten incline dumbbell bench press and as many chest dips as you can manage in two minutes. After a two minute pause you should repeat the exercises and then repeat a second time.

Once that has been completed you can do ten tricep extensions followed by ten one arm dumbbell extensions, (for each arm) and another ten standard tricep extension. Again, this should be repeated twice.

Finally a barbell front raise and a dumbbell lateral raise should be completed; ideally twelve of each. Again this exercise should be repeated twice to show the maximum effect.

Although specific weights are mentioned it is possible to use an alternative. Anything which is heavy but can be held in one hand will do for the majority of these exercises; even a tool box stuffed with tools or rocks can provide the necessary resistance.

3. Interval training Session

Interval training has been credited with improving general fitness and muscle building for many years. This is because you are forcing your body to explode into short bursts of actions. This is much more tiring and demanding of your muscles; it makes them work harder and grow faster to ensure they are capable of the necessary burst of speed.

This is a great method of improving muscle whilst completing almost any physical exercise; you could go running, swilling, in the gym or even take part in strongman style competitions. Simply choose your preferred sport and then select your interval. There is no right or wrong when trying this method; it is what works best for you and your needs. For example you could have a fifteen second sprint, literally running as fast as you possibly can. You will then need to rest for a minute or two before you do the same sprint. There is no limit to the number of times that you can repeat the sprint; until you are physically incapable is one possibility! Alternatively you could do a five minute burst and then break for five or ten minutes. The key is to recover completely before you start again. This will ensure every exercise has your maximum effort and reduce the chance of you becoming injured.

If you are new to this type of training it is worth noting that you may not be able to go flat out even for fifteen seconds. This should not be an issue; simply work harder than you normally would for those fifteen seconds; it will get easier and you will get stronger.

4. Plyometric workout

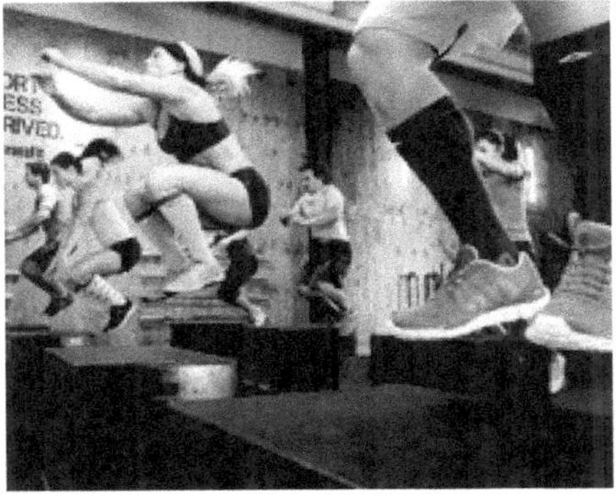

This is an extension of the interval training technique. Each of the exercises in this type of routine are designed to provide an instant load on your body; this stretches the muscles and is instantly reversed by contracting them. All of the exercise which is classed as plyometric are fast paced. This includes things like springing or rope skipping. Even throwing a ball hard and fast can count; such as baseball or football.

There are a range of exercises to undertake; the best way to start plyometric training is by engaging in something simple like skipping or hurdling. Even jumping onto a low box can be a good starting point. The more advanced you become the better you will be able to do these exercises and you can move to burpee pull-ups or even repetitive box jumping.

These sudden exercises create an oxygen deficiency in your body and enable you to burn large amounts of fat in a short space of time. You will find that you only have to do several jumps to start feeling out of breath. It is essential to focus on your form and complete each exercise properly; if you do not then you increase the likelihood of injury. It is also important to work different muscle groups each time you exercise. This will prevent muscle fatigue and injury.

5. *Cardio Boxing*

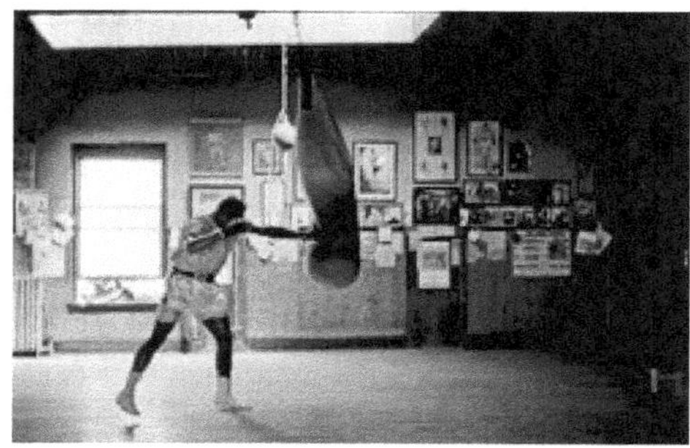

This workout will focus on your reactions and on building core muscles. A strong core will enable you to undertake a variety of challenges which might otherwise seem impossible.

As the name suggests this workout is focused on boxing. It has been shown to be a great form of exercise and an excellent way of building muscle as well as having some fun!

A simple version of this involves using a punch bag at home, although you may find more benefit with a real sparring partner. The trick to creating a good workout is to mix a variety of high intensity moves and keep your heart pumping hard at all times. This will ensure you receive the benefit of a cardio workout and increase your stamina as well as your ability to fight.

Chapter 3 – Five Advanced Level Workouts

Once you have undertaken a variety of these exercises for some time your level of fitness and muscular tone should be dramatically improving and you will be ready to move to the next level. By this stage you should have noticed a difference in your general fitness and you may even have had comments regarding your body and the improvement that is now visible. Advanced workouts reflect this level of fitness and the strength now present in your body. In fact, the best way to proceed when you reach this level is to mix a variety of the different exercise routines together. Your workout can still be completed within half an hour at home; or anywhere you have the time spare. Ideally you should mix a variety of workouts from the beginner levels, intermediate and the advanced level. The more you mix up the workouts the harder your body will have to work. It will also not become so accustomed to a specific workout regime that it no longer has any effect.

The following workouts are high intensity and are very rewarding.

1. *The Muscle Builder*

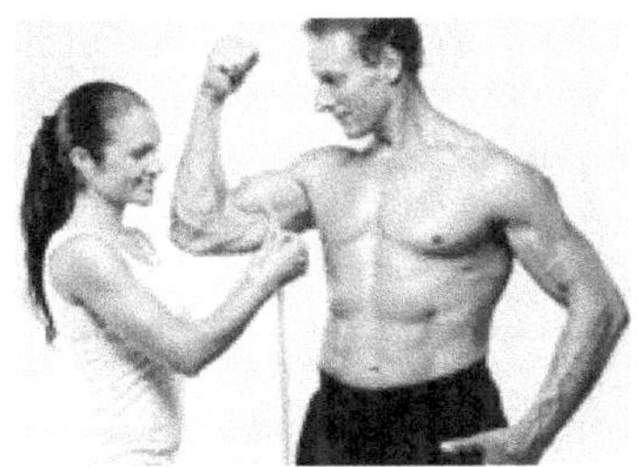

http://ephedrixfacts.com/wp-content/uploads/2014/12/musclebuilding1_600x450.jpg

This intensive routine will test your fitness level and improve your overall tone as well as helping you to stay slim. If possible you should repeat the following exercises three times:

Squats – lasting thirty seconds, followed by push ups on dumbbells or similar elevation item. This should be followed by thirty seconds of lunges and a fast sprint for thirty seconds.

You can then complete another thirty seconds of squats and forty seconds of dumbbell chest presses; followed by more elevated press ups and then forty seconds of pull-ups; using a door frame of pull up bar.

Another thirty second sprint gets you ready for another round of squats (forty seconds); whilst holding kettlebell weights; or a barbell if you have one. You will then need to complete forty seconds of dumbbell rows and one minute worth of push ups. To finish you should complete forty seconds of lunges; switching sides as you do so and then forty seconds of burpees.

Once you have completed this be sure to rest for a few minutes before you start the routine again. Even when you are ready for advanced workouts; this one is physically demanding.

2. *Bodyweight workout*

You have already experienced some of the bodyweight exercise regime, however the following routine is more intense and physically demanding. It is designed to improve your physique even further and get you ready for any challenge. In fact, it is recommended that you have been completing strength training and other exercises regularly for at least a year before you attempt the following routine:

You must warm up before any exercise and it is recommended you complete a five minute walk or jog to help you warm up your muscles.

You will need to start with the jump lunge. This involves starting in the familiar lunge position and pushing off into a jump; both legs will be straight and int he air. You can then land back into the lunge position. This needs to be repeated at least ten times.

The next move is your basic push up; however as you go up you will need to push yourself higher than usual; this will provide you with the opportunity to clap your hands together before lowering yourself back down.

You can then move onto a single leg bridge. Start on your back with one foot flat on the floor and your knee bent. The other one should be in the air, at ninety degrees from your waist and with the knee bent at ninety degrees. Simply lift your hips from the ground and lift as high as you can; whilst maintain your posture. Repeat this at least ten times.

You will then be ready to complete the side plank. Simple face sideways and keep one foot on the ground and one arm. Then lift the other arm above you and one leg; effectively creating a star. Hold the pose for several seconds and then lower. Again you will need to repeat the pose at least ten times; once completed you should repeat all the exercise at least once, preferably twice and then warm down slowly.

3. *Alternative Bodyweight Workout*

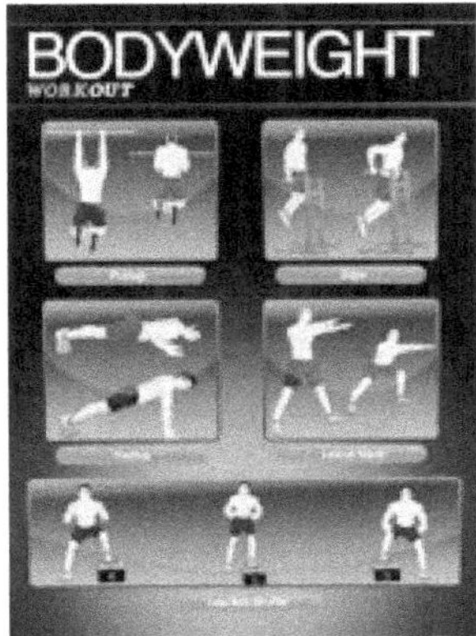

http://www.freefitness24.com/download/Workout%20Posters/bodyweight-workout.jpg

This offers the same benefits as the workout above but is in a different format.

It starts with the squat, as in the previous workout. However, in this one when you jump you need to spin before landing back into the squat position. The idea is to have your back to where you just jumped; effectively turning one hundred and eighty degrees whilst performing a squat. You should do at least ten of these.

You can follow this exercise with a balancing plank. This involves adopting the standard plank position with both toes and both elbows on the floor. Then lift one arm in the air, superman style and lift the opposite leg. You should hold this pose for at least thirty seconds before lowering yourself back to the floor. Then, you should repeat the plank two more times.

Next you get to be Superman! Lie on the floor and lift your arms, head and legs into the air. Hold the pose for five seconds then slowly lower them back to the floor. Repeat this exercise at least ten times.

You can then take a two minute break before repeating every step of the exercise; attempting to do one more of each exercise than you did on the first attempt. Finally you will be able to repeat this one more time to reach the thirty second marks.

4. *High Intensity Workout*

This is designed to increase your stamina as well as your core muscles. Each exercise must be completed twice; every exercise is strenuous and considered to be high impact. You must be at the right level to try this; if you are not you are likely to cause yourself an injury.

As this routine is exceptionally demanding it is best to only complete it once or twice a week.

Once you have warmed up you can start by completing twenty seconds of lateral hops. This means jumping as high as you can from left to right and back as though hopping with both legs.

You can then progress to completing some push up jacks. This is your standard push up position and then jumping into a star position whilst remaining facing the ground. They should last for twenty seconds followed by twenty seconds worth of lunges; when you spring between left and right lunges.

Next is the traditional push up but you need to push your body into the air so that your hands leave the ground. This should lead into hopping on one leg for twenty seconds. You can then switch legs and continue your hoping before repeating your hands in the air push ups.

Next, lie on your back and place a football on your feet; which are together. Lift your feet up ninety degrees and grab the ball with your hands. Repeat these ten times and then twist from side to side; holding the top part of your body still as you do ten on each side. The next step is from a squatting position to jump and turn before landing in the squatting position again and dropping straight into a sideways push up; repeat ten times.

You can then repeat the entire workout once after a one minute rest.

5. *Military Workout*

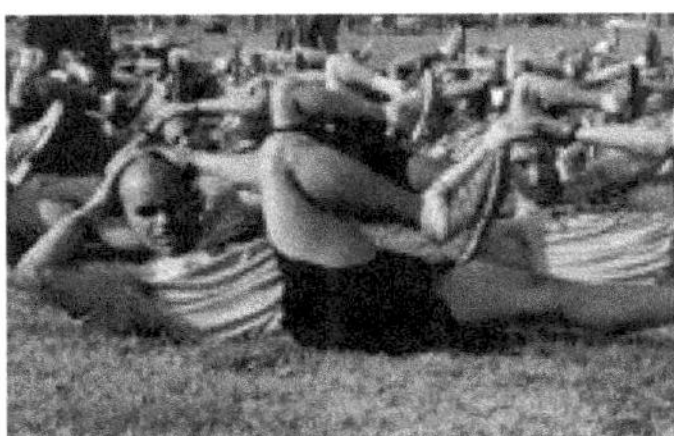

http://imageso4.military.com/media/military-fitness/tradoc-revises-army-physical-fitness-test-image.jpg

This workout will test your entire body and is not one which should be undertaken lightly. You must already be in good physical shape to be able to complete it properly.

To start you will need to complete ten push ups, ten crunches, ten wide stance push ups, another ten crunches followed by ten tricep push ups and ten left crunches and ten right crunches. You should then repeat this routine ten times. You can then move onto your leg exercises and perform twenty squats, twenty crunches, ten lunches on each leg, another twenty crunches and twenty calf raises. Repeat these exercises five times. Next you will need to run one mile in approximately seven minutes, follow this with a quarter mile sprint in less than one hundred seconds and then jog another quarter mile. Alternatively you can swim or even walk this stage but you will need to adjust the activity accordingly.

This seemingly simple workout will test the limits of your endurance!

Conclusion

It is possible to undertake almost any exercise in the comfort of your own home or even when you are out and about. Whist there is an abundance of specialist equipment in many gyms; it can often be more rewarding and more challenging to use the items which are in the natural environment. This will often push your body to greater limits than the artificial props and will certainly help to build your stamina as well as muscle definition.

However, before you undertake any exercise program, it is essential to know what it is you hope to get from the different regimes. There is a big difference between slimming down and improving your muscle tone as compared to building your muscles and becoming as big as possible. The latter needs the gym and all the heavy weight lifting gear. Someone who is simply interested in improving their fitness and the general look of their body can achieve a great deal through the workouts described in this book.

There are many benefits to starting and sticking to a regular workout schedule; the majority of these revolve around an increased level of fitness and a corresponding increase in the level of energy you have available. As already mentioned the best approach to these exercises is to mix and match them as much as possible. Your body will become accustomed to the same work out and it will have much less effect than it originally did. By switching between the different types of exercise you are likely to lose more weight and improve your muscle definition.

The secret to consistently training and improving your muscular physique is in variety. You can choose exercises which target specific muscle groups and mix them with the workouts described in this book. Equally you can choose to use different parts of each workout routine. Providing you recognize your own limits you can utilize any of the techniques described. Pushing your limits is an acceptable and necessary part of training, but going too far will cause an injury and ruin your training for a considerable length of time. Finding the balance involves changing your routine every time you become comfortable with a set of exercises. You may also find it beneficial to train with a friend; this will help both of you to stick to the training and a little competition can help to improve the speed of your results. Above all, you should always warm up and warm down before and after exercising; this will dramatically reduce the chance of injuring yourself.

FREE Bonus Reminder

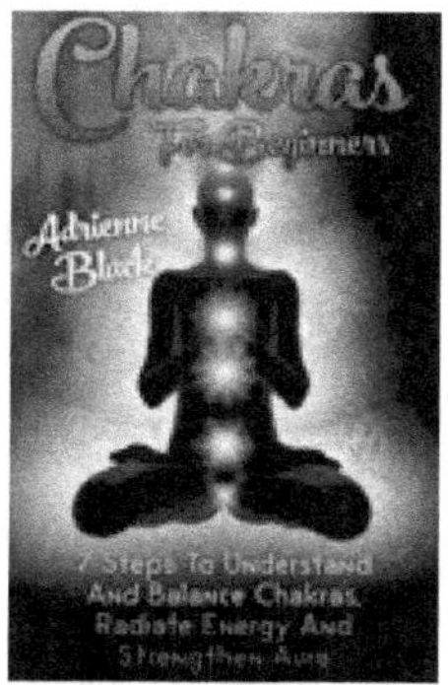

If you have not grabbed it yet, please go ahead and download your special bonus E book *"Chakras for Beginners. 7 Steps To Understand And Balance Chakras, Radiate Energy, And Strengthen Aura"*.

Simply Click the Button Below

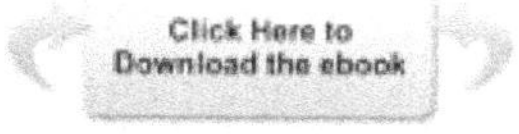

OR Go to This Page

http://lifehacksworld.com/free

BONUS #2: More Free & Discounted Books & Products

Do you want to receive more Free/Discounted Books or Products?

We have a mailing list where we send out our new Books or Products when they go free or with a discount on Amazon. Click on the link below to sign up for Free & Discount Book & Product Promotions.

=> Sign Up for Free & Discount Book & Product Promotions <=

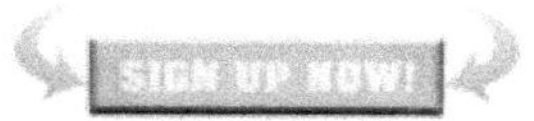

OR Go to this URL

http://zbit.ly/1WBb1Ek